<u>***Welcome To Your Self-care Journey.***</u>

Self-care is a crucial aspect of our well-being, and it is especially important for women, who often juggle multiple roles and responsibilities. Taking care of ourselves allows us to show up as our best selves in all areas of our lives, and it is an act of self-love and respect.

In this book, you will find practical tips, activities, and self-care practices that you can incorporate into your daily routine. We will explore various dimensions of self-care, including physical, emotional, mental, and spiritual well-being. We will also delve into the intersection of self-care and social justice, as self-care is not just about pampering ourselves, but also about building resilience, advocating for our needs, and creating a more equitable and compassionate world.

I hope this book serves as a helpful resource for you on your self-care journey. Remember, self-care is not a luxury, but a necessity. It is an ongoing process that requires us to be mindful, attentive, and kind to ourselves. So let's embrace self-care and nurture our whole selves!
*Self-Care Worksheets and Journal Prompts at the end of every chapter.

Table of Contents

Dear Beautiful Soul,

Welcome to a journey of self-discovery, empowerment, and unapologetic self-love. This book is crafted with you in mind—the resilient, powerful, and extraordinary Black woman navigating the intricate tapestry of life. In a world that often demands more than it gives, self-care becomes not just a luxury but a revolutionary act, a radical declaration that affirms your worthiness of joy, healing, and holistic well-being.

As Black women, our identities are multi-faceted, weaving together threads of strength, beauty, and cultural richness. We are the nurturers, the trailblazers, the caregivers, and the backbone of communities. Yet, in the midst of pouring into others, we may inadvertently neglect the most important person—ourselves.

This book is a testament to the belief that self-care is not selfish; it is a necessary foundation for living a fulfilling and purposeful life. It acknowledges the unique challenges and triumphs that come with being a Black woman and provides a sanctuary where you can explore, reflect, and embrace the fullness of who you are.

Chapter 1: Cultivating a Mindful Mindset

In the hustle and bustle of our daily lives, it's easy to lose ourselves in the chaos, forgetting to cherish the present moment. For Black women, the weight of multiple roles and responsibilities can be especially demanding, making it crucial to intentionally cultivate a mindful mindset. Mindfulness isn't just a buzzword; it's a transformative practice that allows us to embrace the beauty of each moment and reconnect with our inner selves.

Understanding Mindfulness

At its core, mindfulness is the art of being fully present—engaging in the here and now without judgment. It's about immersing ourselves in the richness of our experiences, whether they are moments of joy, challenges, or the simple beauty of everyday life. As Black women, our stories are deeply rooted in resilience, and mindfulness becomes a tool to honor and nurture that resilience.

Mindful Breathing Exercises

Let's begin with the breath—a powerful anchor to the present moment. Find a quiet space, sit comfortably, and close your eyes. Inhale deeply, feeling the air fill your lungs. Exhale slowly, releasing any tension or stress. Repeat this process, focusing solely on your breath. Notice the rise and fall of your chest. In this simple act, you are embracing mindfulness, grounding yourself in the present.

Mindfulness is not reserved for meditation sessions alone; it can be seamlessly woven into your daily activities. Whether you're sipping a cup of tea, walking in nature, or engaging in routine tasks, invite your awareness to fully participate in the experience. Feel the warmth of the sun on your skin, savor the flavors of your meal, and appreciate the beauty in the ordinary.

In the journey of cultivating a mindful mindset, self-compassion is key. Be gentle with yourself; allow room for imperfections and growth. Remember, mindfulness is not about perfection but about awareness and acceptance.

As Black women, our journey to mindfulness is a celebration of our strength, a recognition of our worthiness, and a reclaiming of our mental and emotional well-being. In the subsequent chapters, we will explore additional mindfulness practices and delve into ways to integrate this transformative mindset into various aspects of our lives.

Join me in embracing the power of mindfulness—a practice that not only enriches our individual lives but also contributes to the collective well-being of our communities.

Let's begin with the breath—a powerful anchor to the present moment. Find a quiet space, sit comfortably, and close your eyes. Inhale deeply, feeling the air fill your lungs. Exhale slowly, releasing any tension or stress. Repeat this process, focusing solely on your breath. Notice the rise and fall of your chest. In this simple act, you are embracing mindfulness, grounding yourself in the present.

Incorporating Mindfulness into Daily Life

Mindfulness is not reserved for meditation sessions alone; it can be seamlessly woven into your daily activities. Whether you're sipping a cup of tea, walking in nature, or engaging in routine tasks, invite your awareness to fully participate in the experience. Feel the warmth of the sun on your skin, savor the flavors of your meal, and appreciate the beauty in the ordinary.

In the journey of cultivating a mindful mindset, self-compassion is key. Be gentle with yourself; allow room for imperfections and growth. Remember, mindfulness is not about perfection but about awareness and acceptance.

As Black women, our journey to mindfulness is a celebration of our strength, a recognition of our worthiness, and a reclaiming of our mental and emotional well-being. In the subsequent chapters, we will explore additional mindfulness practices and delve into ways to integrate this transformative mindset into various aspects of our lives.

Join me in embracing the power of mindfulness—a practice that not only enriches our individual lives but also contributes to the collective well-being of our communities.

Reflection Prompt:

"What are three things that you are grateful for right now?"

<u>**Mindful Journaling Exercise:**</u>

"Write about a recent situation where you felt stressed or overwhelmed. What thoughts or actions might help you approach this kind of situation more mindfully next time?"

Practical Action:

"Practice mindful breathing for five minutes today. Write down how you felt before and after. What changes did you notice?"

Chapter 2: Nurturing Your Body

In the beautiful tapestry of our existence, our bodies are the vessels through which we navigate the world. As Black women, our bodies carry the weight of history, strength, and resilience. Nurturing our physical well-being is an essential aspect of self-care—a practice that honors the sacred connection between our bodies and our overall sense of wellness.

Holistic Health for Black Women

Holistic health recognizes the interconnectedness of our physical, mental, and spiritual well-being. As Black women, our bodies may carry the imprints of generational experiences, and prioritizing holistic health allows us to address both the visible and invisible dimensions of our well-being. Begin by acknowledging the wisdom embedded in your body—the stories it tells, the strength it embodies, and the resilience it signifies.

Fitness and Exercise Tips

Exercise is not just about sculpting our bodies; it's a celebration of movement and vitality. Explore activities that bring you joy, whether it's dancing, walking, yoga, or any form of physical expression. Engaging in regular exercise not only promotes physical health but also contributes to mental clarity and emotional well-being. Make it a ritual to move your body with intention and gratitude.

Journaling for Emotional Release

One of the most powerful tools for emotional wellness is journaling. Putting your thoughts on paper allows you to release bottled-up emotions. Get yourself a journal where you can freely express your feelings—both the good and the bad. Let your pen flow without censorship. Journaling is a safe space, and it offers a beautiful release that will leave you feeling lighter.

Building Resilience

Resilience doesn't mean being unaffected by life's challenges; it means rising despite them. Black women have an incredible reservoir of resilience, but it doesn't come without emotional strain. Building resilience involves allowing yourself to be vulnerable and accepting support when you need it. Therapy, sister circles, and safe spaces where you can speak your truth are invaluable for processing emotions and fostering emotional well-being.

Take time to feel, heal, and build resilience with love and compassion. Your emotions are valid, and your emotional wellness is key to thriving.

Healthy Eating Habits

The nourishment we provide to our bodies is a reflection of self-love. Embrace a balanced and nourishing diet that supports your unique needs. Explore the vibrant tapestry of African and diasporic cuisines, rich in flavors and cultural significance. Be mindful of the foods that energize and sustain you, cultivating a harmonious relationship with your body through mindful eating practices. Nurturing your body is not about conforming to external standards but about honoring your body's unique needs and rhythms.

Listen to your body's cues, prioritize rest, and seek professional guidance when needed. In doing so, you affirm the importance of your well-being, acknowledging that self-care encompasses the physical vessel that carries you through life.

As Black women, embracing our bodies is an act of rebellion against societal norms that may seek to diminish our worth. In the subsequent chapters, we will continue to explore practices that celebrate and uplift the physical essence of who we are. Join me on this journey of body positivity, holistic health, and the celebration of the extraordinary vessel that is your body.

Chapter 3: Embracing Your Emotions

Our emotions are part of what makes us beautifully human, but for many Black women, we've been conditioned to be "strong" at all costs. We hold it together through adversity, pain, and challenges. While strength is a virtue, so is vulnerability. It's time we embrace all our emotions without judgment. Self-care begins when we honor every feeling—whether it's joy, sadness, anger, or love—as a valid and necessary part of our journey.

The Importance of Emotional Wellness

Emotional wellness isn't about being happy all the time; it's about understanding and managing your emotions in healthy ways. Your emotions are messengers. When you feel overwhelmed, anxious, or frustrated, it's your body's way of telling you that something needs attention. Pay attention to the signals your emotions send, and don't be afraid to give yourself the space to feel. Emotional wellness also means embracing joy unapologetically. Society often tells Black women that our joy should be diminished or secondary to our struggles. But sis, your joy is revolutionary. Celebrate your wins, bask in your accomplishments, and give yourself permission to be soft and carefree.

Journaling for Emotional Release

<u>Chapter 3: Embracing Your Emotions Activities</u>

<u>Reflection Prompt:</u>

"What emotions have you been avoiding or suppressing lately? How can you make space to feel and process them?"

<u>**Journaling Exercise:**</u>

"Write a letter to yourself expressing compassion and understanding for a difficult emotion you've recently felt. Use this letter to remind yourself that it's okay to feel whatever you're feeling."

<u>Emotional Wellness Tracker:</u>

"Track your emotions for the next three days. Write down how you felt throughout the day, what triggered those emotions, and any ways you were able to practice self-compassion."

<u>**Chapter 4: Celebrating Black Beauty**</u>

Black beauty is a powerful affirmation of our uniqueness. But let's be honest—living in a world that often places Eurocentric beauty standards on a pedestal can make us feel like we're not enough. It's time to reject that narrative. Your melanin, your curls, your curves, your features—they are all worthy of celebration.

Loving Your Natural Self

Sis, your natural beauty is magic. Whether you wear your hair in braids, an afro, locs, or straightened, know that your beauty is your own definition. Loving yourself starts with rejecting societal ideals that try to box you in. Let your beauty shine in its authenticity. Embrace your natural hair, your skin tone, and all the features that make you uniquely you.

Skincare and Haircare Rituals

Caring for your skin and hair is more than just aesthetics—it's a ritual of self-love. Establish a skincare routine that nourishes and celebrates the beauty of your melanin. From deep cleansing to moisturizing with rich oils, taking time for your skin is an act of self-care that honors your natural beauty.

When it comes to hair, experiment with styles that make you feel empowered. Invest in haircare products that nourish your scalp and strands. Whether you're protective styling, rocking your natural curls, or switching it up with a weave or wig, remember that how you wear your hair is your choice and no one else's.

Chapter 4: Celebrating Black Beauty Activities

Beauty Reflection:

"List five things you love about your physical appearance and why they make you unique. How does celebrating your beauty make you feel?"

<u>**Journaling Exercise:**</u>

"Reflect on how societal beauty standards have affected your self-image. Write about how you are learning to embrace your own beauty, regardless of external pressures."

<u>**Body and Beauty Care Goals:**</u>

"What small steps can you take this week to enhance your beauty rituals?

Example: Create a skincare routine, invest in a new hair product, or wear a bold

lip color that makes you feel confident."

Chapter 5: Fostering Sisterhood and Community

Black women thrive in community. Our bonds are a source of strength, healing, and joy. Sisterhood is a form of self-care—it's a place where we find support, love, and acceptance without judgment. Our connections with other Black women allow us to recharge and share our stories in ways only we can understand.

The Power of Sisterhood

Sisterhood means showing up for one another. It's the deep, soulful connections we build with other Black women who walk the same path and understand the same struggles. Invest in these relationships. Whether it's calling a friend to check in, attending a women's group, or gathering with sisters for a Sunday brunch, these moments of connection are powerful acts of self-care. Lean into sisterhood; it's a wellspring of love and support.

Building Supportive Networks

Building a support system is essential to your self-care journey. Create spaces where you feel safe, uplifted, and valued. Surround yourself with women who pour into you and empower you to be your best self. Celebrate their successes as much as you celebrate your own. A supportive network is built on mutual respect, love, and care.

__Community Engagement for Well-Being__

Self-care extends beyond ourselves—it's about uplifting our communities. Engage in community events, volunteer, and advocate for causes that matter to you. When we take care of our communities, we also nurture ourselves. We are each other's keepers, and being actively involved in the betterment of our people is an expression of love, solidarity, and care.

Chapter 5: Fostering Sisterhood and Community Activities

Reflection Prompt:

"Who are the women in your life who support and uplift you? Write down how they contribute to your well-being and how you can nurture those relationships."

<u>Journaling Exercise:</u>

"What does sisterhood mean to you? How do you feel when you're surrounded by women who understand and support you?"

<u>**Actionable Step:**</u>

"Reach out to one of your closest sisters this week. Let her know how much she means to you, and plan a time to connect. Whether it's a coffee date or a phone call, nurturing these bonds is part of your self-care."

Chapter 6: Balancing Multiple Roles

Many of us wear multiple hats: we're caregivers, professionals, friends, daughters, partners, and more. While these roles bring fulfillment, they can also create stress and overwhelm if we don't find balance. Achieving balance doesn't mean doing it all perfectly—it means knowing when to pause, recharge, and set boundaries.

Navigating Work-Life Balance

As Black women, we often feel like we have to work twice as hard to prove our worth. But sis, you are already worthy. Prioritize balance by setting boundaries between your work and personal life. Don't be afraid to say no to extra work or responsibilities that drain you. You deserve time to rest, recharge, and focus on your personal needs.

Managing Family and Personal Time

Family is at the core of our culture, and as Black women, we often carry the weight of caregiving for both immediate and extended family. While taking care of loved ones is important, make sure you're not neglecting yourself in the process. Carve out time just for you—whether it's a quiet evening with a good book, a solo trip, or a bubble bath. Your time is valuable, and you deserve moments of peace.

Setting Boundaries

The key to balance is setting boundaries—something that can be challenging when we're used to giving so much of ourselves. But remember: boundaries are a form of self-respect. They allow you to protect your time, energy, and mental well-being. Practice saying "no" without guilt, and create space for the things that truly nourish you.

<u>Chapter 6: Balancing Multiple Roles Activities</u>

<u>Reflection Prompt:</u>

"Think about the different roles you play in life (e.g., mother, partner, employee). How do you feel about the balance between these roles? Are there any that are taking up more space than you'd like?"

<u>**Setting Boundaries Exercise:**</u>

"Write down one boundary you'd like to set in your work, personal life, or with family. How will this boundary help you feel more balanced and less overwhelmed?"

<u>**Balance Planner:**</u>

"Create a self-care schedule for the week. Include at least three activities that are just for you—whether it's reading a book, exercising, or taking a nap. Prioritize your own needs just as you do for others."

Chapter 7: Spiritual Self-Care

Spirituality is a core part of who we are as Black women. It's the foundation that guides us, comforts us, and connects us to something greater than ourselves. Spiritual self-care is about nurturing your soul, feeding your spirit, and aligning with your higher purpose.

Connecting with Your Spirituality

Whether you follow a specific faith tradition or define spirituality on your own terms, connect with what brings you peace and purpose. Prayer, meditation, reading sacred texts, or simply spending time in nature can help you cultivate a deeper spiritual connection. Whatever practices resonate with your spirit, make time for them in your self-care routine.

Creating Sacred Spaces

A sacred space doesn't have to be elaborate; it just needs to be intentional. Dedicate a corner of your home for reflection, prayer, or meditation. Light candles, burn incense, or use calming essential oils to create an atmosphere of peace. This is your space to retreat, recharge, and connect with your inner self.

Rituals and Practices for Inner Peace

Incorporate spiritual rituals into your daily routine. It could be as simple as beginning your day with gratitude, journaling about your intentions, or engaging in evening meditation. Rituals provide a sense of grounding and remind us of our spiritual connection, even in the busiest of days.

Chapter 7: Spiritual Self-Care Activities

Spiritual Reflection:

"What practices or beliefs make you feel spiritually grounded and connected? How can you incorporate more of these into your daily routine?"

<u>**Journaling Exercise:**</u>

"Write about a time when you felt deeply connected to something bigger than yourself—whether it was during prayer, meditation, or in nature. How did this experience impact your sense of peace and purpose?"

<u>**Daily Gratitude Ritual:**</u>

"For the next week, start each morning by listing three things you're grateful for. This simple practice will help you cultivate a mindset of abundance and spiritual alignment."

Chapter 8: Social Justice and Self-Care

As Black women, our existence is inherently political. Navigating systemic racism, sexism, and inequality can take a toll on our mental, emotional, and physical health. While self-care is deeply personal, it is also a form of resistance—a radical act of prioritizing our well-being in a society that often devalues it.

Intersectionality and Well-Being

Black women sit at the intersection of multiple identities—race, gender, class, and more. These intersections shape our experiences, and it's important to recognize how they impact our well-being. Acknowledging these intersections allows us to be more intentional about the type of self-care we need and deserve.

Advocating for Change

Advocating for social justice and self-care go hand in hand. Whether you're protesting in the streets, supporting Black-owned businesses, or educating others about systemic injustices, know that your voice matters. Activism can be emotionally exhausting, so remember to care for yourself in the process. Rest when you need to, and recharge in community spaces where you feel supported.

Self-Care as a Form of Activism

Taking care of ourselves in a world that seeks to oppress us is an act of defiance. It's saying, "I am worthy of rest, love, and care." Whether you're engaging in activism or simply living your life authentically, self-care is a way to reclaim your power and assert your right to joy and well-being.

Chapter 8: Social Justice and Self-Care Activities

Reflection Prompt:

"How has your experience with social justice movements impacted your personal well-being? In what ways have you practiced self-care while advocating for change?"

<u>**Journaling Exercise:**</u>

"Write about a cause that is close to your heart. How can you balance your involvement in activism with taking care of your mental, emotional, and physical health?"

<u>**Social Justice Action Plan:**</u>

"Create a self-care strategy for when you're involved in activism. What practices will help you stay grounded? How will you recharge after participating in events or protests?"

<u>**Chapter 9: Releasing Perfectionism and Embracing Your True Self**</u>

Perfectionism can be a heavy burden that many of us carry, often unknowingly. As Black women, the pressure to be perfect may stem from society's unrealistic expectations, cultural pressures, or the desire to prove ourselves in spaces that were not designed with us in mind. But here's the truth: Perfectionism is not your friend, and it doesn't serve your higher self. In fact, it can be one of the biggest barriers to authentic self-care.

In this chapter, we'll explore how to release perfectionism and embrace your true self—imperfections and all. Because your worth isn't tied to being flawless, it's tied to being real, to showing up as you are, and to loving yourself unconditionally.

<u>**Recognizing Perfectionism**</u>

Perfectionism can sneak into our lives in subtle ways. Maybe you find yourself avoiding certain tasks or projects because you don't want to make a mistake. Or perhaps you feel like no matter how much you accomplish, it's never enough. These are signs that perfectionism may be affecting you.

Perfectionism often comes from a place of fear—fear of failure, fear of judgment, fear of not being "good enough." But the truth is, perfection is an illusion. No one is perfect, and chasing after perfection only leaves us exhausted, anxious, and disconnected from ourselves.

The Power of Vulnerability One of the most powerful ways to release perfectionism is to embrace vulnerability. Being vulnerable means showing up as you are, without hiding behind a facade of perfection. It means allowing yourself to make mistakes, to be human, and to learn from your experiences.

Vulnerability is not weakness; it's strength. When you allow yourself to be vulnerable, you open yourself up to deeper connections with others and with yourself. You also give yourself permission to grow, to evolve, and to accept that you are already enough.

Embracing Your True Self At the core of releasing perfectionism is the practice of embracing your true self. This means accepting your flaws, quirks, and imperfections as part of what makes you unique and beautiful. It means understanding that you don't have to be perfect to be worthy of love, respect, and care.

When you stop striving for perfection and start embracing who you are, you free yourself from the constant pressure to perform. You create space for self-compassion, for growth, and for joy.

So, let's make a commitment to let go of perfectionism. You are already enough, just as you are. And you deserve to live a life where you can show up authentically, without the weight of unrealistic expectations.

<u>**Chapter 9: Releasing Perfectionism and Embracing Your True Self Activities**</u>

<u>**Reflection Prompt:**</u>

"In what areas of your life do you feel the most pressure to be perfect? How does perfectionism show up for you, and how does it make you feel?"

<u>**Vulnerability Journaling Exercise:**</u>

Write about a time when you allowed yourself to be vulnerable. How did it feel to show up authentically, without trying to be perfect? What did you learn from that experience?"

<u>**Practical Action:**</u>

"This week, practice letting go of perfectionism in one area of your life. Whether it's at work, in a relationship, or in your self-care routine, give yourself permission to make mistakes and be imperfect. Write about how it feels and any challenges you encounter."

Chapter 10: Sustaining Your Self-Care Practice

Self-care is not a one-time act or something you check off a to-do list. It's a practice—a lifelong journey of nurturing your mind, body, and spirit. In this final chapter, we'll focus on how to sustain your self-care practice, ensuring that it becomes an integral part of your life, rather than something you only turn to in times of stress.

Consistency is key when it comes to self-care. Just like any habit, the more you prioritize and practice self-care, the more it will become a natural and essential part of your routine. But sustaining self-care isn't about being rigid or strict with yourself.
It's about flexibility, balance, and listening to what your body and soul need at any given moment.

Creating a Self-Care Plan One of the best ways to ensure that self-care remains a consistent part of your life is to create a self-care plan. A self-care plan helps you outline the practices and rituals that nurture you and make you feel whole. It's a personal roadmap for maintaining your well-being, even when life gets busy or challenging.

<u>*When creating your self-care plan, consider the following:*</u>

- **<u>Daily Practices:</u>** What are small, daily acts of self-care that you can commit to? This could be something as simple as taking a few minutes to breathe deeply, drinking water, or stretching.

- **<u>Weekly Rituals:</u>** What are the bigger self-care practices that you can incorporate weekly? This might include journaling, exercising, or spending time with loved ones.

- **<u>Monthly Check-Ins:</u>** How can you check in with yourself regularly to assess how you're feeling and what adjustments you need to make to your self-care routine?

<u>Adapting to Life's Changes</u>

Life is constantly changing, and so too will your self-care needs. There will be times when you need more rest, more connection, or more solitude. There will also be times when you feel energized and ready to take on new challenges. The key to sustaining your self-care practice is to adapt it to the ebb and flow of life.

Give yourself permission to change your self-care routine as needed. Listen to your body and your inner wisdom. Some weeks, your self-care might look like bubble baths and long naps; other weeks, it might look like setting boundaries and saying no to commitments that drain your energy.

The Importance of Community As you continue on your self-care journey, remember that you don't have to do it alone. Surround yourself with a supportive community of friends, family, or even online spaces where you can share your experiences and receive encouragement. Community can be a powerful source of inspiration and accountability when it comes to maintaining your self-care.

By sustaining your self-care practice, you're making a commitment to prioritize your well-being every day. This is a lifelong journey, and it's one worth investing in. You deserve to be cared for, nurtured, and loved—by yourself, first and foremost.

Chapter 10: Sustaining Your Self-Care Practice Activities

Reflection Prompt:

"What does sustainable self-care look like for you? How can you incorporate self-care into your daily, weekly, and monthly routines?"

<u>**Self-Care Plan Creation:**</u>

"Create your personal self-care plan. List your daily, weekly, and monthly self-care practices. Think about what actions nurture you the most and how you can prioritize those in your schedule."

<u>Self-Care As Liberation</u>

Dear sister,

self-care is not just a trend; it's a lifelong journey of liberation, healing, and empowerment. As Black women, we are worthy of every ounce of care, love, and attention we give ourselves. This book is only the beginning of a journey that invites you to continually pour into yourself, honor your body and soul, and reclaim your joy.

You are magic. You are resilient. and most importantly, you are enough. As you move forward, remember that self-care is not a destination; it's a practice. It's a commitment to show up for yourself every single day, no matter what. May you carry the lessons from these chapters with you, and may you always remember that taking care of yourself is your birthright.

With love and light,

♥